CALIFORNIA
MEDICAL
MARIJUANA
DISPENSARIES
2014

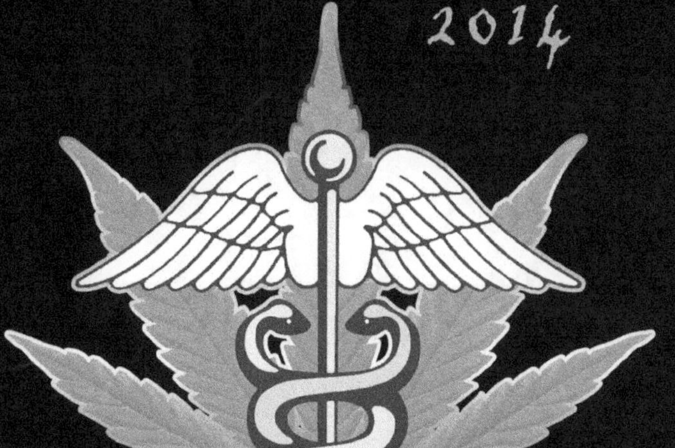

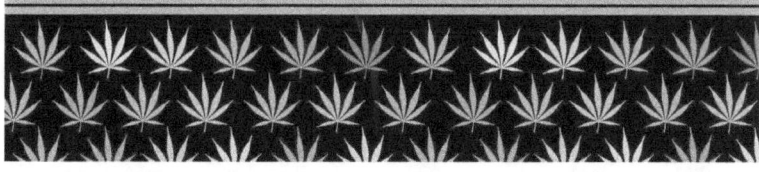

CALIFORNIA MEDICAL MARIJUANA
DISPENSARIES 2014
Most Popular Cannabis Dispensaries in California

© Harry F. Engholm, 2014
© E.G.P. Editorial, 2014

Printed in USA.

ISBN-13: 978-1502372307
ISBN-10: 1502372304

CALIFORNIA MEDICAL MARIJUANA DISPENSARIES 2014

Most Popular Cannabis Dispensaries in California

*This directory is dedicated to California Business Owners and Managers
who provide the experience that the patients enjoy.
Thanks you very much for all that you do and thank for being the "People Choice".*

*Thanks to everyone that posts their reviews online and
the amazing reviews sites that make our life easier.*

*The places listed in this book are the most positively reviewed
and recommended by doctors and patients.*

*Thank you for your time and enjoy the directory that is
designed with patients in mind!*

CALIFORNIA
MEDICAL
MARIJUANA
DISPENSARIES

#1
Exhale Med Center
Cannabis Dispensary
Area: West Hollywood
Address: 980 N La Cienega Blvd
Los Angeles, CA 90069
Phone: (424) 279-9497

#2
ECMM
Medical Evaluations
Area: Culver City
Address: 13347 W Washington Blvd
Los Angeles, CA 90066
Phone: (424) 835-4137

#3
Nirvana Dispensary
Cannabis Dispensary
Area: East Hollywood
Address: 4511 W Sunset Blvd
Los Angeles, CA 90027
Phone: (323) 663-4444

#4
California Compassionate Care Network
Cannabis Dispensary
Area: North Hollywood
Address: 4720 Vineland Ave
Los Angeles, CA 91602
Phone: (818) 980-6337

#5
HHC Hollywood Hills Collective
Cannabis Dispensary
Area: Hollywood Hills
Address: 3324 Barham Blvd
Los Angeles, CA 90068
Phone: (323) 380-6207

#6
Club La Brea Medical Marijuana Dispensary
Cannabis Dispensary
Area: Mid-Wilshire
Address: 351 S La Brea Ave
Los Angeles, CA 90036
Phone: (323) 674-9867

#7
California Caregivers Alliance
Cannabis Dispensary
Area: Silver Lake
Address: 2815 W Sunset Blvd
Los Angeles, CA 90026
Phone: (213) 353-0100

#8
Cornerstone Research Collective
Cannabis Dispensary
Area: Eagle Rock
Address: 2551 Colorado Blvd
Los Angeles, CA 90041
Phone: (323) 259-8933

#9
Green Path Collective
Cannabis Dispensary
Area: Mid-City
Address: 8707 Venice Blvd
Los Angeles, CA 90034
Phone: (424) 298-8580

#10
CCSC
Cannabis Dispensary
Area: Fairfax
Address: 7324 Melrose Ave
Los Angeles, CA 90046
Phone: (323) 930-0550

#11
Precision Medical Caregivers
Cannabis Dispensary
Area: Koreatown, Wilshire Center
Address: 3913 W 6 Street
Los Angeles, CA 90020
Phone: (213) 382-7971

#12
TGE
Cannabis Dispensary
Area: Beverly Grove
Address: 7948 W 3rd St
Los Angeles, CA 90048
Phone: (323) 782-8022

#13
House Of Dank
Cannabis Dispensary
Area: Pico-Union
Address: 2253 W Pico Blvd
Los Angeles, CA 90006
Phone: (213) 252-8220

#14
Grace Medical
Cannabis Dispensary
Area: Sawtelle
Address: 12320 Pico Blvd
Los Angeles, CA 90064
Phone: (310) 826-2592

#15
1437 N La Brea Collective
Cannabis Dispensary
Area: Hollywood
Address: 1437 N La Brea Ave
Los Angeles, CA 90028
Phone: (818) 588-1185

#16
HERB
Cannabis Dispensary
Area: Downtown
Address: 500 S Main St
Los Angeles, CA 90014
Phone: (844) 437-2213

#17
Hollywood High Grade
Cannabis Dispensary
Area: Hollywood
Address: 7051 B Santa Monica Blvd
Los Angeles, CA 90038
Phone: (323) 536-9133

#18
Downtown Patient Group
Cannabis Dispensary
Area: Downtown
Address: 1753 S Hill St
Los Angeles, CA 90015
Phone: (213) 747-3386

#19
Hyperion Healing
Cannabis Dispensary
Area: Los Feliz
Address: 1913 Hyperion Ave
Los Angeles, CA 90027
Phone: (323) 953-1913

#20
Medstar
Cannabis Dispensary
Area: Pico-Robertson
Address: 1155 S Robertson Blvd
Los Angeles, CA 90035
Phone: (310) 385-5860

#21
California Herbal Remedie
Cannabis Dispensary
Area: El Sereno
Address: 5468 Valley Blvd.
Los Angeles, CA 90032
Phone: (323) 342-9110

#22
Greenhouse Herbal Center
Cannabis Dispensary
Area: East Hollywood
Address: 5224 Hollywood Blvd
Los Angeles, CA 90027
Phone: (323) 666-2591

#23
Mr Greens Collective
Cannabis Dispensary
Area: Silver Lake
Address: 3740 W Sunset Blvd
Los Angeles, CA 90026
Phone: (323) 913-0668

#24
Clean Green LAX
Cannabis Dispensary
Area: Westchester
Address: 8338 Lincoln Blvd
Los Angeles, CA 90045
Phone: (310) 421-1446

#25
La Brea Collective
Cannabis Dispensary
Area: Mid-Wilshire
Address: 5057 W Pico Blvd
Los Angeles, CA 90019
Phone: (323) 424-3908

#26
Sunset Junction Organic Medicine
Cannabis Dispensary
Area: Silver Lake
Address: 4017 W Sunset Blvd
Los Angeles, CA 90029
Phone: (323) 660-0655

#27
Pico Patient Wellness
Cannabis Dispensary
Area: Pico-Union
Address: 2273 W. Pico Blvd.
Los Angeles, CA 90006
Phone: (213) 674-7388

#28
Laxcc
Cannabis Dispensary
Area: Westchester
Address: 8332 Lincoln Blvd
Los Angeles, CA 90045
Phone: (310) 439-9176

#29
Koreatown Collective
Cannabis Dispensary
Area: Fairfax
Address: 7382 Melrose Ave
Los Angeles, CA 90046
Phone: (323) 951-9513

#30
Speed Weed
Cannabis Dispensary
Area: Hollywood Hills
Address: 3400 Cahuenga Blvd W
Los Angeles, CA 90068
Phone: (888) 860-8472

#31
Dabs on Wheels
Cannabis Dispensary
Area: Highland Park
Address:
Los Angeles, CA 90042
Phone: (323) 257-6337

#32
Natural Ways Always Caregivers
Cannabis Dispensary
Area: Palms
Address: 10006 1/2 National Blvd
Los Angeles, CA 90034
Phone: (310) 837-7004

#33
The Farmacy Westwood
Cannabis Dispensary
Area: Westwood, UCLA
Address: 1001 Gayley Ave
Los Angeles, CA 90024
Phone: (310) 208-0820

#34
Charity Collective
Cannabis Dispensary
Area: Hollywood Hills
Address:
Los Angeles, CA 90068
Phone: (818) 397-7707

#35
Venice Collective
Cannabis Dispensary
Area: Mar Vista
Address: 12581 Venice Blvd
Los Angeles, CA 90066
Phone: (310) 437-0308

#36
CANNAcierge
Cannabis Dispensary
Area: Downtown
Address: 503 W 7th St
Los Angeles, CA 90017
Phone: (818) 693-6060

#37
Studio Pharms Collective
Cannabis Dispensary
Area: Studio City
Address: 12427 Ventura Blvd
Los Angeles, CA 91604
Phone: (818) 980-2100

#38
Pacific Organic
Cannabis Dispensary
Area: Chinatown
Address:
Los Angeles, CA 90012
Phone: (424) 240-8768

#39
The OG Spot
Cannabis Dispensary
Area: Westwood
Address: 1779 Westwood Blvd
Los Angeles, CA 90024
Phone: (323) 484-3645

#40
Hollyweed Dispensary
Cannabis Dispensary
Area: Hollywood
Address: 1607 N El Centro Ave
Los Angeles, CA 90028
Phone: (323) 469-9873

#41
Green Street Junction Collective
Cannabis Dispensary
Area: Los Feliz
Address: 4514 Hollywood Blvd
Los Angeles, CA 90027
Phone: (323) 644-0500

#42
Organic Caregivers
Cannabis Dispensary
Area: West Los Angeles
Address: 2249 Westwood Blvd
Los Angeles, CA 90064
Phone: (310) 270-2482

#43
City of Angels Wellness Center
Cannabis Dispensary
Area: Hollywood
Address: 6435 W Sunset Blvd
Los Angeles, CA 90028
Phone: (323) 466-2295

#44
The Doctor's - Hollywood - Medical Marijuana Evaluations
Cannabis Dispensary
Area: Hollywood
Address: 1439 N Highland Blvd
Los Angeles, CA 90028
Phone: (323) 463-5000

#45
Westwood Village Collective
Cannabis Dispensary
Area: Westwood, UCLA
Address: 10966 Le Conte Ave
Los Angeles, CA 90024
Phone: (310) 208-4254

#46
Studio City Caregivers
Cannabis Dispensary
Area: Studio City
Address: 3625 Cahuenga Blvd
Los Angeles, CA 90068
Phone: (323) 850-1847

#47
Greener Pastures Collective
Cannabis Dispensary
Area: Pico-Robertson
Address: 1101 S Robertson Blvd
Los Angeles, CA 90035
Phone: (310) 550-6993

#48
Sunset Herbal Corner
Cannabis Dispensary
Area: Hollywood
Address: 7225 W Sunset Blvd
Los Angeles, CA 90046
Phone: (323) 851-5554

#49
NoHo
Cannabis Dispensary
Area: North Hollywood
Address: 5656 Cahuenga Blvd
Los Angeles, CA 91601
Phone: (818) 762-8962

#50
Kind for Cures
Cannabis Dispensary
Area: Palms
Address: 9850 Exposition Blvd
Los Angeles, CA 90034
Phone: (310) 836-5463

#51
Medical Marijuana Card Doctor Hollywood Easy Dispensary
Cannabis Dispensary
Area: Hollywood
Address: 7127 Sunset Blvd
Los Angeles, CA 90046
Phone: (323) 790-4983

#52
The Clinik
Cannabis Dispensary
Area: Hollywood
Address: 7101 W Sunset Blvd
Los Angeles, CA 90046
Phone: (323) 798-5243

#53
LA Confidential Caregivers
Cannabis Dispensary
Area: Fairfax
Address: 7263 Melrose Ave
Los Angeles, CA 90046
Phone: (323) 424-4157

#54
Rx Caregiving
Cannabis Dispensary
Area: Atwater Village
Address: 4600 Sperry St
Los Angeles, CA 90039
Phone: (818) 241-6033

#55
Buds On Melrose
Cannabis Dispensary
Area: Fairfax
Address: 7418 Melrose Ave
Los Angeles, CA 90046
Phone: (323) 272-4972

#56
Downtown Natural Caregiviers
Cannabis Dispensary
Area: Downtown
Address: 312 S Wall St
Los Angeles, CA 90013
Phone: (213) 625-0301

#57
Westlake Collective
Cannabis Dispensary
Area: Pico-Union
Address: 1675 W 11th St
Los Angeles, CA 90015
Phone: (424) 777-8099

#58
City of Angels AHC
Cannabis Dispensary
Area: East Hollywood
Address: 4877 Melrose Ave
Los Angeles, CA 90004
Phone: (323) 464-2222

#59
The Bud Stop Collective
Cannabis Dispensary
Area: Valley Glen
Address: 12439 Victory Blvd
Los Angeles, CA 91606
Phone: (818) 200-6792

#60
420 Evaluations MD
Cannabis Dispensary
Area: Leimert Park
Address: 4343 Crenshaw Blvd
Los Angeles, CA 90008
Phone: (323) 696-0071

#61
Green Earth Collective
Cannabis Dispensary
Area: Highland Park
Address: 5045 York Blvd
Los Angeles, CA 90042
Phone: (323) 982-9042

#62
Grand Daddy Purp
Cannabis Dispensary
Area: University Park
Address: 2626 S Figueroa St
Los Angeles, CA 90007
Phone: (213) 746-6535

#63
215 Pharmacy
Cannabis Dispensary
Area: Mid-City
Address: 6134 W Pico Blvd
Los Angeles, CA 90035
Phone: (323) 413-2493

#64
SL Caregivers
Cannabis Dispensary
Area: Harvard Heights
Address: 1126 S Western Ave
Los Angeles, CA 90015
Phone: (213) 747-1752

#65
Downtown Direct Caregivers
Cannabis Dispensary
Area: Westlake
Address: 3219 Beverly Blvd
Los Angeles, CA 90057
Phone: (213) 427-3727

#66
TQ Healing
Cannabis Dispensary
Area: Echo Park
Address: 2623 W Sunset Blvd
Los Angeles, CA 90026
Phone: (213) 973-6369

#67
Evergreen Collective
Cannabis Dispensary
Area: Hollywood
Address: 1606 N Gower St
Los Angeles, CA 90028
Phone: (323) 466-2100

#68
Greener By Nature Collective
Cannabis Dispensary
Area: Brentwood
Address: 11919 Wilshire Blvd
Los Angeles, CA 90025
Phone: (323) 515-4400

#69
Washington Boulevard Collective
Cannabis Dispensary
Area: Mid-City
Address: 5024 Washington Blvd
Los Angeles, CA 90016
Phone: (323) 931-2697

#70
The Coughy Shop
Cannabis Dispensary
Area: Mount Washington
Address: N San Fernando Rd
Los Angeles, CA 90065
Phone: (323) 550-1533

#71
Golden Coast Organics
Cannabis Dispensary
Area: Harvard Park
Address: 1427 W Florence Ave
Los Angeles, CA 90001
Phone: (818) 579-6358

#72
Super Green Bear
Cannabis Dispensary
Area: Historic South Central
Address: 350 E Jefferson
Los Angeles, CA 90011
Phone: (213) 744-9765

#73
Kenmore Medical Collective
Cannabis Dispensary
Area: Koreatown
Address: 261 S Kenmore Ave
Los Angeles, CA 90004
Phone: (213) 384-3881

#74
Nature's Wonder Caregivers
Cannabis Dispensary
Area: Arlington Heights
Address: 4143 W Pico Blvd
Los Angeles, CA 90019
Phone: (323) 731-5874

#75
Venezia Discount Collective
Cannabis Dispensary
Area: Boyle Heights
Address: 3018 Washington Blvd
Los Angeles, CA 90023
Phone: (310) 827-3800

#76
Mecca Natural Medicine
Cannabis Dispensary
Area: Mid-City
Address: 5650 W Washington Blvd
Los Angeles, CA 90016
Phone: (323) 937-0299

#77
Harmony Herbal Healing
Cannabis Dispensary
Area: Echo Park
Address: 2501 W Sunset Blvd
Los Angeles, CA 90026
Phone: (213) 529-4647

#78
Stargate Collective
Cannabis Dispensary
Area: Los Feliz
Address: 1903 Hyperion Ave
Los Angeles, CA 90027
Phone: (323) 665-4867

#79
LA Kush Hemporium
Cannabis Dispensary
Area: Mid-City
Address: 5113 W Pico Blvd
Los Angeles, CA 90019
Phone: (323) 935-0808

#80
The Holistic Pharmacy
Cannabis Dispensary
Area: Pico-Union
Address: 2649 W Pico Blvd
Los Angeles, CA 90006
Phone: (213) 427-9280

#81
Hi Point
Cannabis Dispensary
Area: Carthay
Address: 5925 W Pico Blvd
Los Angeles, CA 90035
Phone: (323) 932-1723

#82
Canna Health Caregivers
Cannabis Dispensary
Area: Mid-City
Address: 5658 W Pico Blvd
Los Angeles, CA 90019
Phone: (323) 932-0370

#83
Medical Caregivers Association
Cannabis Dispensary
Area: Lincoln Heights
Address: 1804 N Broadway
Los Angeles, CA 90031
Phone: (323) 551-5874

#84
Asclepius
Cannabis Dispensary
Area: Fairfax
Address: 7381 Melrose Ave
Los Angeles, CA 90046
Phone: (323) 951-9513

#85
Downtown Collective
Cannabis Dispensary
Area: Downtown
Address: 1600 S. Hill St
Los Angeles, CA 90015
Phone: (213) 746-5420

#86
Advanced Natural Medical Center/Dispensary
Cannabis Dispensary
Area: East Hollywood
Address: 330 N Western Ave
Los Angeles, CA 90004
Phone: (323) 836-0420

#87
Fly Delivery
Cannabis Dispensary
Area: Glendale
Address:
Los Angeles, CA 91206
Phone: (323) 905-4359

#88
Bluegate Collective
Cannabis Dispensary
Area: Boyle Heights
Address: 3428 Whittier Blvd
Los Angeles, CA 90023
Phone: (323) 263-3009

#89
420 Med Evaluation
Cannabis Dispensary
Area: Mid-City
Address: 2622 S Robertson Blvd
Los Angeles, CA 90034
Phone: (310) 237-1277

#90
Los Angeles Patient's Association
Cannabis Dispensary
Area: Downtown
Address: 106 E 17th St
Los Angeles, CA 90015
Phone: (213) 747-7397

#91
Buds 4 Less Wellness
Cannabis Dispensary
Area: Florence
Address: 5923 S Broadway
Los Angeles, CA 90003
Phone: (424) 777-8099

#92
Zen Garden
Cannabis Dispensary
Area: North Hollywood
Address: 4702 Vineland Ave
Los Angeles, CA 91602
Phone: (424) 666-9990

#93
Community Earth Grown Meds
Cannabis Dispensary
Area: Gramercy Park
Address: 7609 1/2 S Western Ave
Los Angeles, CA 90047
Phone: (323) 759-9871

#94
Mary Janes's Collective
Cannabis Dispensary
Area: East Hollywood
Address: 4901 Melrose Ave
Los Angeles, CA 90004
Phone: (323) 466-6636

#95
SoCal 420 Doctor Medical Marijuana
Cannabis Dispensary
Area: Mid-City
Address: 2126 S La Brea
Los Angeles, CA 90016
Phone: (888) 999-6951

#96
Elevation Wellness
Cannabis Dispensary
Area: Valley Glen
Address: 13122 Sherman Way
Los Angeles, CA 91605
Phone: (818) 765-5933

#97
ASR Affordable Solutions for Relief
Cannabis Dispensary
Area: Silver Lake
Address: 608 N Hoover St
Los Angeles, CA 90004
Phone: (323) 667-9667

#98
Field of Greens
Cannabis Dispensary
Area: Mid-City
Address: 5226 W Pico Blvd
Los Angeles, CA 90019
Phone: (323) 424-3050

#99
Soto Street Collective
Cannabis Dispensary
Area: Boyle Heights
Address: 1260 Soto St
Los Angeles, CA 90023
Phone: (323) 262-8280

#100
The Lucky Spot
Cannabis Dispensary
Area: Echo Park
Address: 1306 N Glendale Blvd
Los Angeles, CA 90026
Phone: (213) 407-0941

#101
LA Natural
Cannabis Dispensary
Area: Downtown
Address: 1319 S Los Angeles
Los Angeles, CA 90015
Phone: (213) 745-5500

#102
Green Cross Medical Dispensary
Cannabis Dispensary
Area: Vermont-Slauson
Address: 5832 S Vermont Ave
Los Angeles, CA 90044
Phone: (323) 750-7354

#103
Colorado Healing Center
Cannabis Dispensary
Area: Glassell Park
Address: 4110 1/2 Verdugo Rd
Los Angeles, CA 90065
Phone: (323) 474-6024

#104
215 Caregivers
Cannabis Dispensary
Area: Lincoln Heights
Address: 3119 N Main St
Los Angeles, CA 90031
Phone: (323) 227-5874

#105
420MD Evaluation
Medical Evaluations
Address: 603 E 121th St
Los Angeles, CA 90059
Phone: (323) 696-0071

#106
VHC Club
Cannabis Dispensary
Area: Palms
Address: 10955 Venice Blvd
Los Angeles, CA 90034
Phone: (310) 837-5100

#107
Kelly's Collective
Cannabis Dispensary
Area: Pico-Robertson
Address: 8638 W Pico Blvd
Los Angeles, CA 90035
Phone: (310) 854-5874

#108
**Beach Enlightenment And
Compassionate Healing**
Cannabis Dispensary
Area: Playa del Rey
Address: 310 Culver Blvd
Los Angeles, CA 90293
Phone: (310) 821-4420

#109
Spectrum
Cannabis Dispensary
Area: Koreatown
Address: 3567 W 3rd St
Los Angeles, CA 90020
Phone: (213) 273-3764

#110
Amsterdam Mart
Cannabis Dispensary
Area: East Hollywood
Address: 4718 Fountain Ave
Los Angeles, CA 90027
Phone: (310) 256-9959

#111
Hot Zone Medical
Cannabis Dispensary
Area: Downtown
Address: 1612 S Hill St
Los Angeles, CA 90015
Phone: (213) 765-6099

#112
Organic Treatment Center
Cannabis Dispensary
Area: Hollywood
Address: 1119 N Hudson Ave
Los Angeles, CA 90038
Phone: (323) 464-6404

#113
Angel City Caregivers
Cannabis Dispensary
Area: Pico-Union
Address: 1314 Venice Blvd
Los Angeles, CA 90006
Phone: (213) 986-6099

#114
Share Luck Collective
Cannabis Dispensary
Area: Lincoln Heights
Address: 1804 N Bdwy
Los Angeles, CA 90031
Phone: (323) 551-5874

#115
Medcity
Cannabis Dispensary
Area: Mid-City
Address: 5140 W Washington Blvd
Los Angeles, CA 90016
Phone: (323) 939-0001

#116
Red Eye Society
Cannabis Dispensary
Area: Koreatown, Wilshire Center
Address: 737 S Vermont
Los Angeles, CA 90005
Phone: (213) 381-3420

#117
La Brea Caregivers
Cannabis Dispensary
Area: Mid-Wilshire
Address: 1188 S La Brea Ave
Los Angeles, CA 90019
Phone: (323) 549-0400

#118
Medical Advisory Center
Cannabis Dispensary
Area: Koreatown, Wilshire Center
Address: 4311 Wilshire Blvd
Los Angeles, CA 90010
Phone: (323) 965-0420

#119
215 Collective
Cannabis Dispensary
Area: East Hollywood
Address: 4534 Fountain Ave
Los Angeles, CA 90029
Phone: (323) 669-1885

#120
Green Royalty Collective
Cannabis Dispensary
Area: Hollywood
Address: 6025 Santa Monica Blvd
Los Angeles, CA 90038
Phone: (323) 546-3333

#121
Cali Natural Collective
Cannabis Dispensary
Area: Hollywood
Address: 744 N La Brea Ave
Los Angeles, CA 90038
Phone: (323) 939-9102

#122
Ultimate New Age Care Inc
Cannabis Dispensary
Area: Fairfax
Address: 7280 Melrose Ave
Los Angeles, CA 90046
Phone: (323) 939-9339

#123
Fly Delivery
Cannabis Dispensary
Area: Atwater Village
Address:
Los Angeles, CA 90039
Phone: (323) 905-4359

#124
Artists Collective
Cannabis Dispensary
Area: Hollywood Hills
Address:
Los Angeles, CA 90068
Phone: (818) 397-7707

#125
Southern California Collective
Cannabis Dispensary
Area: Mar Vista
Address: 12583 Venice Blvd
Los Angeles, CA 90066
Phone: (310) 806-0067

#126
Sherman Wellness
Cannabis Dispensary
Area: Van Nuys
Address: 7218 Van Nuys Blvd
Los Angeles, CA 91405
Phone: (818) 826-3434

#127
The Green Elephant
Cannabis Dispensary
Area: Leimert Park
Address: 4309 Crenshaw Blvd
Los Angeles, CA 90008
Phone: (213) 426-8160

#128
Lab Rats Mobile Service
Cannabis Dispensary
Area: Koreatown, Wilshire Center
Address: Greater Los Angeles
Los Angeles, CA 90005
Phone: (323) 973-8090

#129
Medical Marijuana Evaluation Center
Cannabis Dispensary
Area: Eagle Rock
Address: 4344 Eagle Rock Blvd
Los Angeles, CA 90041
Phone: (323) 474-6702

#130
Herbal Healing Center
Cannabis Dispensary
Area: Carthay
Address: 1051 S Fairfax Ave
Los Angeles, CA 90019
Phone: (323) 934-4314

#131
Hemp Factory
Cannabis Dispensary
Area: Hollywood
Address: 6250 santa monica Blvd
Los Angeles, CA 90038
Phone: (323) 960-0772

#132
Westwood THC
Cannabis Dispensary
Area: Westwood
Address: 1561 Westwood Blvd
Los Angeles, CA 90024
Phone: (424) 248-3132

#133
Downtown Discount Center
Cannabis Dispensary
Area: Westlake
Address: 1123 W 7th St
Los Angeles, CA 90017
Phone: (213) 309-3331

#134
Southern Roots Collective
Cannabis Dispensary
Area: Downtown
Address: 653 S Main St
Los Angeles, CA 90014
Phone: (323) 667-8665

#135
LA Wonderland Caregivers
Cannabis Dispensary
Area: Mid-City
Address: 4410 W Pico Blvd
Los Angeles, CA 90019
Phone: (323) 936-4410

#136
Exhale Hollywood
Cannabis Dispensary
Area: Hollywood
Address: 1724 N Cahuenga
Los Angeles, CA 90028

#137
Medical Marijuana Doctors
Cannabis Dispensary
Area: Pico-Union
Address: 2267 W Pico Blvd
Los Angeles, CA 90006
Phone: (323) 251-0058

#138
Alternameds
Cannabis Dispensary
Area: Sunland
Address: 8517 Foothill Blvd
Los Angeles, CA 91040
Phone: (818) 951-4555

#139
Hoyland Group
Cannabis Dispensary
Area: Van Nuys
Address: 13521 Sherman Way
Los Angeles, CA 91405
Phone: (818) 994-0600

#140
Premium Pacific Collective
Cannabis Dispensary
Area: Westchester
Address: 8332 Lincoln Blvd
Los Angeles, CA 90045
Phone: (310) 439-9176

#141
Aardvarks Co-Op
Cannabis Dispensary
Area: Mid-Wilshire
Address: 5597 Pico Blvd
Los Angeles, CA 90019
Phone: (323) 424-4754

#142
Green Mile Collective
Cannabis Dispensary
Area: Mid-City
Address: 4512 1/2 W Pico Blvd
Los Angeles, CA 90019
Phone: (323) 692-0048

#143
Natural Remedies Caregivers
Cannabis Dispensary
Area: Hollywood
Address: 927 1/2 N Western
Los Angeles, CA 90029
Phone: (323) 871-9500

#144
La Luna Collective Lounge
Cannabis Dispensary
Area: Fairfax
Address: 7406 Melrose Ave
Los Angeles, CA 90046
Phone: (323) 655-9333

#145
Downtown Holistic Center
Cannabis Dispensary
Area: Echo Park
Address: 1160 Glendale Blvd
Los Angeles, CA 90026
Phone: (213) 787-3101

#146
Kind Meds
Cannabis Dispensary
Area: Encino
Address: 17049 Ventura Blvd
Los Angeles, CA 91316
Phone: (818) 783-2768

#147
House Of Sky
Cannabis Dispensary
Area: Van Nuys
Address: 7902 Woodley Ave
Los Angeles, CA 91406

#148
Eden Caregivers
Cannabis Dispensary
Area: Downtown
Address: 718 S Hill St
Los Angeles, CA 90014
Phone: (213) 627-1004

#149
Berkeley Dispensary
Cannabis Dispensary
Area: Hollywood
Address: 6430 Selma Ave
Los Angeles, CA 90028
Phone: (323) 848-4650

#150
OtherSide Health Management
Cannabis Dispensary
Area: Hollywood
Address: 6115 Selma Ave
Los Angeles, CA 90028
Phone: (323) 871-2488

#151
The Famous Joint
Cannabis Dispensary
Area: Pacoima
Address: 13120 Van Nuys Blvd
Los Angeles, CA 91331
Phone: (818) 899-7300

#152
Mission Hills Organic
Cannabis Dispensary
Area: Mission Hills
Address: 10736 Sepulveda Blvd
Los Angeles, CA 91345
Phone: (818) 639-6027

#153
Green Light Delivery
Cannabis Dispensary
Area: Larchmont
Address:
Los Angeles, CA 91356
Phone: (424) 888-4204

#154
The Green Doctors
Cannabis Dispensary
Area: Venice
Address: 2007 Ocean Front Walk
Los Angeles, CA 90291
Phone: (310) 985-2233

#155
Pico Healing Center
Cannabis Dispensary
Area: Mid-Wilshire
Address: 5597 W Pico Blvd
Los Angeles, CA 90019
Phone: (323) 215-8849

#156
The Green Easy
Cannabis Dispensary
Area: Beverly Grove
Address: 8311 Beverly Blvd
Los Angeles, CA 90048
Phone: (323) 424-3035

#157
THC Exposé
Cannabis Dispensary
Area: Downtown
Address: 1201 S Figueroa St.
Los Angeles, CA 90015

#158
CC&M Organic
Cannabis Dispensary
Area: Reseda
Address: 7131 Lindley Ave
Los Angeles, CA 91335
Phone: (818) 708-1700

#159
Organics: Herbal Nutrition Center
Cannabis Dispensary
Area: Pico-Robertson
Address: 1435 S La Cienega Blvd
Los Angeles, CA 90035
Phone: (310) 657-4148

#160
BHPC
Cannabis Dispensary
Area: Lincoln Heights
Address: 1812 N Broadway
Los Angeles, CA 90031
Phone: (323) 454-7863

#161
Fresh Collective
Cannabis Dispensary
Area: Hollywood
Address: 1523 N La Brea
Los Angeles, CA 90028
Phone: (323) 603-7531

#162
**The Doctors - Los Angeles
Medical Cannabis Evaluations**
Cannabis Dispensary
Area: East Hollywood
Address: 1155 N Vermont Ave
Los Angeles, CA 90029
Phone: (213) 446-5462

#163
Organic Medirex Consultations
Cannabis Dispensary
Area: North Hollywood
Address: 11335 Magnolia Blvd North
Hollywood, CA 91601
Phone: (818) 505-8805

#164
West Coast Collective
Cannabis Dispensary
Area: Boyle Heights
Address: 1500 Esperanza St.
Los Angeles, CA 90023
Phone: (323) 266-7116

#165
Pure Decision Association
Cannabis Dispensary
Area: Hollywood
Address: 6122 Santa Monica Blvd
Los Angeles, CA 90038
Phone: (818) 288-0422

#166
Friendly Meds
Cannabis Dispensary
Area: East Hollywood
Address: 5415 Santa Monica
Los Angeles, CA 90029
Phone: (323) 229-6127

#167
Wellness Earth Energy Dispensary
Cannabis Dispensary
Area: Studio City
Address: 11557 Ventura Blvd
Studio City, CA 91604
Phone: (818) 980-2266

#168
GEM Health Group
Cannabis Dispensary
Area: Tujunga
Address: 7502 Foothill Blvd.
Los Angeles, CA 91042
Phone: (818) 353-1070

#169
The Dragon Collective
Cannabis Dispensary
Area: Koreatown, Wilshire Center
Address: 3977 W 6th St
Los Angeles, CA 90017
Phone: (213) 529-4016

#170
420 Green Street
Cannabis Dispensary
Area: Beverly Grove
Address:
Los Angeles, CA 90048
Phone: (310) 801-9447

#171
Cool Calm Collective
Cannabis Dispensary
Area: Sherman Oaks
Address: 5658 N Sepulveda
Los Angeles, CA 91403
Phone: (818) 387-6553

#172
Medical Marijuana Doctors
Cannabis Dispensary
Area: Sawtelle
Address: 11320 W Pico Blvd
Los Angeles, CA 90064
Phone: (800) 490-2230

#173
Greenmart
Cannabis Dispensary
Area: Wilmington
Address: 910 W Pacific Coast Hwy
Los Angeles, CA 90744
Phone: (424) 703-3111

#174
**Los Angeles Patients
& Caregivers Group**
Cannabis Dispensary
Area: West Hollywood
Address: 7213 Santa Monica Blvd
West Hollywood, CA 90046
Phone: (323) 882-6033

#175
Strain Genius Labs
Cannabis Dispensary
Area: Downtown
Address: 1600 S Santa Fe Ave
Los Angeles, CA 90021
Phone: (213) 896-0427

#176
The Fountain Of Well Being
Cannabis Dispensary
Area: Los Feliz
Address: 3835 Fountain Ave
Los Angeles, CA 90029
Phone: (323) 662-0900

#177
DOC420
Cannabis Dispensary
Area: Florence
Address: 314 W Florence Ave
Los Angeles, CA 90003
Phone: (818) 794-9269

#178
Eco Rx
Cannabis Dispensary
Area: North Hollywood
Address: 11428 Vanowen St
Los Angeles, CA 91606
Phone: (818) 358-4490

#179
The 710 Club
Cannabis Dispensary
Area: East Hollywood
Address: 874 N Virgil Ave
Los Angeles, CA 90029
Phone: (323) 870-7107

#180
RWC aka The Green Elephant
Cannabis Dispensary
Address: 18527 Roscoe Blvd
Los Angeles, CA 91324

#181
Dollatella Caregivers
Cannabis Dispensary
Area: Sawtelle
Address: 11906 Wilshire Blvd
Los Angeles, CA 90025
Phone: (424) 832-7543

#182
One Love Herbal Collective
Cannabis Dispensary
Area: Palms
Address: 8940 National Blvd
Los Angeles, CA 90034
Phone: (310) 836-6337

#183
Hwood Herb Medical
Cannabis Dispensary
Area: Hollywood
Address: 1103 N El Centro Ave
Los Angeles, CA 90038
Phone: (323) 463-5000

#184
PureLife Alternative Wellness Center
Cannabis Dispensary
Area: Hollywood
Address: 6400 DeLongpre Ave
Los Angeles, CA 90028
Phone: (310) 246-9345

#185
Nature's Natural Cooperative Care
Cannabis Dispensary
Area: Palms
Address: 9021 Exposition Blvd
Los Angeles, CA 90034
Phone: (310) 202-6622

#186
St Andrews Green Dispensary
Cannabis Dispensary
Area: Mid-Wilshire
Address: 659 S La Brea Ave
Los Angeles, CA 90036
Phone: (310) 855-0420

#187
**Hollywood Haute Medicinals
HHM Delivery**
Cannabis Dispensary
Area: Hollywood Hills West
Address: Hollywood Blvd & Vine St
Los Angeles, CA 90046
Phone: (323) 835-5037

#188
Hollywood THC
Cannabis Dispensary
Area: East Hollywood
Address: 5322 W Sunset Blvd
Los Angeles, CA 90027
Phone: (323) 465-9513

#189
Kushmart
Cannabis Dispensary
Area: Downtown
Address: 1343 S Hill St
Los Angeles, CA 90015
Phone: (323) 464-6465

#190
LA Wonderland Caregivers
Cannabis Dispensary
Area: Downtown
Address: 150 Venice Blvd
Los Angeles, CA 90015
Phone: (213) 765-6099

#191
The Happyending Collective
Cannabis Dispensary
Area: Chinatown
Address: 818 North Spring St
Los Angeles, CA 90012
Phone: (213) 625-1124

#192
PharmaJanes
Cannabis Dispensary
Area: Hollywood Hills West
Address:
Los Angeles, CA 90046
Phone: (800) 420-7096

#193
Alternative Medicine Group
Cannabis Dispensary
Area: Brentwood
Address: 641 N Sepulveda Blvd
Los Angeles, CA 90049
Phone: (310) 476-0222

#194
LAHC
Cannabis Dispensary
Area: Westchester
Address: 8621 Bellanca Ave
Los Angeles, CA 90045

#195
Apothecary 420
Cannabis Dispensary
Area: East Hollywood
Address: 330 N Western Ave
Los Angeles, CA 90004
Phone: (323) 836-0420

#196
Associated Patients Collective
Cannabis Dispensary
Area: Toluca Lake
Address: 10714 Riverside Dr
Los Angeles, CA 91602
Phone: (818) 761-1557

#197
Buddha Bar Collective
Cannabis Dispensary
Area: Beverly Grove
Address: 440 1/2 N La Cienega West
Hollywood, CA 90048
Phone: (310) 657-4202

#198
Zen Healing
Cannabis Dispensary
Area: West Hollywood
Address: 8464 Santa Monica Blvd
West Hollywood, CA 90069
Phone: (323) 656-6611

#199
Perennial Holistic Wellness Center
Cannabis Dispensary
Area: Studio City
Address: 11705 Ventura Blvd
Studio City, CA 91604
Phone: (818) 505-3631

#200
Doc420
Cannabis Dispensary
Area: East Hollywood
Address: 4864 Melrose Ave
Los Angeles, CA 90029
Phone: (818) 794-9269

#201
F. G. D'Ambrosio, MD
Cannabis Dispensary
Area: Glassell Park
Address: 4110 1/2 Verdugo Rd
Los Angeles, CA 90065
Phone: (888) 351-7807

#202
The Honey Spot
Cannabis Dispensary
Area: Hollywood
Address: 6775 Santa Monica Blvd
Los Angeles, CA 90038
Phone: (323) 819-8036

#203
Prestige Medical Center
Cannabis Dispensary
Area: West Hollywood
Address: 7855 Santa Monica Blvd West
Hollywood, CA 90046
Phone: (310) 504-1529

#204
Sherman Oaks Organic
Cannabis Dispensary
Area: Sherman Oaks
Address: 13619 Moorpark St
Sherman Oaks, CA 91423
Phone: (818) 616-3122

#205
7333 Shop
Cannabis Dispensary
Area: Canoga Park
Address: 7333 Canoga Ave
Los Angeles, CA 91303
Phone: (818) 703-0399

#206
Kush Collective
Cannabis Dispensary
Area: Mid-Wilshire
Address: 1111 S La Brea Ave
Los Angeles, CA 90019
Phone: (323) 938-5874

#207
The Root Cellar
Cannabis Dispensary
Area: Sherman Oaks
Address: 14517 Ventura Blvd
Sherman Oaks, CA 91403
Phone: (818) 907-1112

#208
Sunset Herbal Corner Weed Shop
Cannabis Dispensary
Area: North Hollywood
Address: 11503 Burbank Blvd
Los Angeles, CA 91601
Phone: (818) 762-2282

#209
Roger A Barnes, MD
Cannabis Dispensary
Area: Pasadena
Address: 1224 E Green St
Pasadena, CA 91106
Phone: (626) 344-7596

#210
Westside Care Givers
Cannabis Dispensary
Area: Mid-City
Address: 2370 S Robertson Blvd
Los Angeles, CA 90034
Phone: (310) 558-0190

#211
Metro Vitality
Cannabis Dispensary
Area: Woodland Hills
Address: Los Angeles, CA 91364
Phone: (818) 471-3684

#212
Buds and Roses Collective
Cannabis Dispensary
Area: Studio City
Address: 13047 Ventura Blvd
Studio City, CA 91604
Phone: (818) 907-8852

#213
Green Angel
Cannabis Dispensary
Area: West Los Angeles
Address: 1716 S Sepulveda Blvd
Los Angeles, CA 90025
Phone: (310) 444-2987

#214
Arts District Healing Center
Cannabis Dispensary
Area: Downtown
Address: 2416 E 8th St
Los Angeles, CA 90021
Phone: (213) 687-9981

#215
Downtown Evaluation Services
Cannabis Dispensary
Area: Pico-Union
Address: 1300 W Olympic Blvd
Los Angeles, CA 90015
Phone: (310) 491-4200

#216
Canna-Centers
Cannabis Dispensary
Address: 15901 Hawthorne Blvd
Lawndale, CA 90260

#217
**The Good Life Marijuana
Delivery Service**
Cannabis Dispensary
Area: Downtown
Address: 506 S Spring St
Los Angeles, CA 90015
Phone: (213) 948-1948

#218
The Higher Path
Cannabis Dispensary
Area: Sherman Oaks
Address: 14080 Ventura Blvd
Sherman Oaks, CA 91423
Phone: (818) 385-1224

#219
Marina Caregivers
Cannabis Dispensary
Area: Del Rey
Address: 13453 Beach Ave
Marina del Rey, CA 90292
Phone: (310) 574-4000

#220
**Medical Marijuana Card Doctor
Studio City Easy Dispensary**
Cannabis Dispensary
Area: Valley Village
Address: 4835 Laurel Canyon Blvd
Los Angeles, CA 91607
Phone: (323) 790-4983

#221
The Greenhouse
Cannabis Dispensary
Area: Sherman Oaks
Address: 5156 Sepulveda Blvd
Sherman Oaks, CA 91403
Phone: (818) 386-1343

#222
Dr Ganja
Cannabis Dispensary
Area: West Hollywood
Address: 7855 Santa Monica Blvd
West Hollywood, CA 90046
Phone: (877) 374-2652

#223
Unified Patient Alliance
Cannabis Dispensary
Area: Sun Valley
Address: 8416 Lankershim Blvd
Los Angeles, CA 91352
Phone: (818) 504-8255

#224
Venice Caregiver Foundation
Cannabis Dispensary
Area: Sun Valley
Address: 8724 Bradley Ave
Los Angeles, CA 91352
Phone: (747) 223-2298

#225
Delta 9 Collective Caregivers
Cannabis Dispensary
Area: Van Nuys
Address: 7648 Van Nuys Blvd.
Van Nuys, CA 91405
Phone: (818) 997-1003

#226
Washington & Western Medical Group
Cannabis Dispensary
Area: Pico-Union
Address: 1876 S Western Ave
Los Angeles, CA 90006
Phone: (323) 373-9456

#227
Valley Herbal Center
Cannabis Dispensary
Area: Sun Valley
Address: 11300 Tuxford St
Los Angeles, CA 91352
Phone: (818) 370-6677

#228
Green Kiss Collective
Cannabis Dispensary
Area: North Hollywood
Address: 6356 Vineland Ave
North Hollywood, CA 91606
Phone: (818) 732-7272

#229
Meds Merchant
Cannabis Dispensary
Area: Sherman Oaks
Address: 14429 Ventura Blvd
Sherman Oaks, CA 91423
Phone: (818) 990-8420

#230
Secret Garden FREE Delivery
Cannabis Dispensary
Area: Santa Monica
Address: Santa Monica, CA 90401
Phone: (310) 697-2611

#231
Holistic Therapeutic Center
Cannabis Dispensary
Area: Valley Village
Address: 12410 Burbank Blvd
Valley Village, CA 91607
Phone: (818) 980-5999

#232
Venice Beach Care Center
Cannabis Dispensary
Area: Venice
Address: 410 Lincoln Blvd
Venice, CA 90291
Phone: (310) 399-4307

#233
YourTree Providers
Cannabis Dispensary
Area: Studio City
Address: 11048 Ventura Blvd
Studio City, CA 91604
Phone: (818) 748-6441

#234
Patients and Caregivers
Cannabis Dispensary
Area: North Hollywood
Address: 6141 Vineland Ave.
North Hollywood, CA 91606
Phone: (818) 588-1307

#235
Venice Medical Center
Cannabis Dispensary
Area: Palms
Address: 9636 Venice Blvd
Culver City, CA 90232
Phone: (424) 603-2133

#236
NoHo Compassionate Caregivers
Cannabis Dispensary
Area: Van Nuys
Address: 14770 Calvert St
Los Angeles, CA 91411
Phone: (818) 902-2155

#237
Green Miracle Healing
Cannabis Dispensary
Area: Sun Valley
Address: 7503 Laurel Canyon Blvd
Los Angeles, CA 91605
Phone: (818) 232-8684

#238
Sherman Oaks Herbal Recommendation
Cannabis Dispensary
Area: Sherman Oaks
Address: 14434 Ventura Blvd
Sherman Oaks, CA 91423
Phone: (818) 387-6202

#239
Los Angeles Valley Caregivers
Cannabis Dispensary
Area: Reseda
Address: 6657 Reseda Blvd
Los Angeles, CA 91335
Phone: (323) 500-1040

#240
The Kind Connect
Cannabis Dispensary
Area: Downtown
Address:
Los Angeles, CA 90013
Phone: (213) 488-2697

#241
Dr Anthony Catipay
Cannabis Dispensary
Area: Sawtelle
Address: 11320 W Pico Blvd
Los Angeles, CA 90064
Phone: (310) 481-4852

#242
Boo-Ku Collective Care
Cannabis Dispensary
Address: 6817 Sepulveda Blvd
Los Angeles, CA 91405

#243
Alternative Herbal Health Services
Cannabis Dispensary
Area: West Hollywood
Address: 7828 Santa Monica Blvd
West Hollywood, CA 90046
Phone: (323) 654-8792

#244
Absolute Healing Collective
Cannabis Dispensary
Area: Woodland Hills
Address: 7041 Owensmouth Ave
Los Angeles, CA 91367
Phone: (626) 200-7843

#245
Little Amsterdam
Cannabis Dispensary
Area: Beverlywood
Address: 2461 S Robertson Blvd
Los Angeles, CA 90034
Phone: (310) 842-4760

#246
VNAS Medical Marijuana Dispensary
Cannabis Dispensary
Area: Van Nuys
Address: 14434 Gilmore St
Van Nuys, CA 91401
Phone: (818) 799-6454

#247
Westside Holistic Remedy
Cannabis Dispensary
Area: West Los Angeles
Address: 2346 Westwood Blvd
Los Angeles, CA 90064
Phone: (310) 441-2800

#248
Green Light Meds
Cannabis Dispensary
Area: Westwood
Address: Santa Monica Blvd & La Cienega
West Hollywood, CA 90069
Phone: (424) 253-5874

#249
Manhattan Beach 420
Cannabis Dispensary
Area: Manhattan Beach
Address: 1601 N Sepulveda
Manhattan Beach, CA 90266
Phone: (855) 768-3278

#250
Kushism
Cannabis Dispensary
Area: Van Nuys
Address: 7555 Woodley Ave
Van Nuys, CA 91406
Phone: (818) 994-3446

#251
Green Goddess Collective
Cannabis Dispensary
Area: Venice
Address: 1716 Main St
Venice, CA 90291
Phone: (310) 396-7770

#252
Sun Valley Caregivers
Cannabis Dispensary
Area: Shadow Hills
Address: 11000 Randall St
Sun Valley, CA 91352
Phone: (818) 504-2661

#253
Canna+Bliss
Cannabis Dispensary
Area: Valley Glen
Address: 7227 Whitsett Ave
Los Angeles, CA 91605
Phone: (818) 982-2236

#254
Harbor Solution Center
Cannabis Dispensary
Area: Harbor City
Address: 23700 S Western Ave
Los Angeles, CA 90710
Phone: (310) 755-9999

#255
The Coffee Joint
Cannabis Dispensary
Area: Encino
Address: 15826 Ventura Blvd
Encino, CA 91436
Phone: (818) 788-1835

#256
La Casa Verde Collective
Cannabis Dispensary
Area: Hollywood Hills West
Address: 1483 Havenhurst Dr.
West Hollywood, CA 90046
Phone: (323) 656-2272

#257
Savon Buds Collective
Cannabis Dispensary
Area: Valley Glen
Address: 5940 Laurel Canyon Blvd
North Hollywood, CA 91607
Phone: (818) 666-5050

#258
La Organics
Cannabis Dispensary
Area: East Hollywood
Address: 5421 Santa Monica Blvd
Los Angeles, CA 90029
Phone: (323) 871-0173

#259
MediCann
Cannabis Dispensary
Area: West Hollywood
Address: 1107 Greenacre Ave
West Hollywood, CA 90046
Phone: (866) 632-6627

#260
Victory Wellness
Cannabis Dispensary
Area: North Hollywood
Address: 5034 Vineland Ave
North Hollywood, CA 91601
Phone: (818) 358-2273

#261
The Medwood Dispensary
Cannabis Dispensary
Address: 302 S Market St
Inglewood, CA 90301

#262
California Alternative Caregivers
Cannabis Dispensary
Area: Venice
Address: 122 S. Lincoln Blvd
Venice, CA 90291
Phone: (877) 219-3809

#263
P.A.S.
Cannabis Dispensary
Area: Pasadena
Address: 638 E Colorado Blvd
Pasadena, CA 91101
Phone: (626) 639-3642

#264
Local 420
Cannabis Dispensary
Area: San Pedro
Address: 600 S Pacific
Los Angeles, CA 90731
Phone: (310) 732-1617

#265
Greenly
Cannabis Dispensary
Area: Del Rey
Address: Marina Del Rey, CA 90292
Phone: (323) 813-6420

#266
Woodvic Medial Care & Dispensary
Cannabis Dispensary
Area: Valley Glen
Address: 13653 Victory Blvd
Van Nuys, CA 91401
Phone: (818) 988-9825

#267
Green Oasis
Cannabis Dispensary
Area: Playa Vista
Address: 11924 W Jefferson Blvd
Culver City, CA 90230
Phone: (310) 397-5700

#268
WHTC
Cannabis Dispensary
Area: Studio City
Address: 3760 Cahuenga Blvd
Studio City, CA 91604
Phone: (818) 980-8338

#269
R and R Collective
Cannabis Dispensary
Area: Studio City
Address: 13205 Ventura Blvd
San Fernando Valley, CA 91604
Phone: (818) 907-9661

#270
A-1 Organic Collective
Cannabis Dispensary
Area: North Hollywood
Address: 10540 Victory Blvd North
Hollywood, CA 91606
Phone: (818) 508-2400

#271
Magic Castle Solutions
Cannabis Dispensary
Area: Sun Valley
Address: 7422 Laurel Canyon Rd
North Hollywood, CA 91605
Phone: (747) 444-8888

#272
Medical Herbs 4 U
Cannabis Dispensary
Area: Reseda
Address: 7122 Reseda Blvd
Reseda, CA 91335
Phone: (818) 666-8080

#273
Smart Collective
Cannabis Dispensary
Area: North Hollywood
Address: 10651 Burbank Blvd
North Hollywood, CA 91601
Phone: (818) 506-4420

#274
The Secret Garden Collective
Cannabis Dispensary
Area: Van Nuys
Address: 5616 1/2 Kester Ave
Van Nuys, CA 91411
Phone: (818) 646-0388

#275
Wild West Collective
Cannabis Dispensary
Area: North Hollywood
Address: 5617 Lankershim Blvd
North Hollywood, CA 91601
Phone: (818) 508-2423

#276
Hazelwood Patients Collective
Cannabis Dispensary
Area: Encino
Address: 17523 Ventura Blvd
Los Angeles, CA 91316
Phone: (818) 793-3972

#277
Green Life Caregivers
Cannabis Dispensary
Area: Tujunga
Address: 7108 Foothill Blvd
Tujunga, CA 91042
Phone: (818) 273-4205

#278
The Spot
Cannabis Dispensary
Area: Hollywood Hills
Address: 3200 Cahuenga Blvd
Los Angeles, CA 90068
Phone: (323) 851-7166

#279
CMG
Cannabis Dispensary
Area: Pasadena
Address: Delivery Service
Pasadena, CA 91106
Phone: (323) 594-0779

#280
Alternative Care Dispensarys
Cannabis Dispensary
Address: 4201 Long Beach Blvd
Long Beach, CA 90807

#281
Starlight Wellness
Cannabis Dispensary
Area: Los Feliz
Address: 1903 Hyperion
Los Angeles, CA 90026
Phone: (323) 545-2200

#282
Mother Nature's Remedy
Cannabis Dispensary
Area: Woodland Hills
Address: 22831 Ventura Blvd
Los Angeles, CA 91364
Phone: (818) 436-2243

#283
Herbalcure
Cannabis Dispensary
Area: Sawtelle
Address: 11318 W Pico Blvd
Los Angeles, CA 90064
Phone: (310) 312-5215

#284
Medical Marijuana Card Center
Cannabis Dispensary
Area: Reseda
Address: 6853 Reseda Blvd
Reseda, CA 91335
Phone: (818) 462-5650

#285
South Gate Herbal Healing Center
Cannabis Dispensary
Address: 13194 Paramount Blvd
South Gate, CA 90280

#286
Oh Gee Remedies
Cannabis Dispensary
Area: Tujunga
Address: 7004 Foothill Blvd
Tujunga, CA 91042
Phone: (818) 951-9991

#287
TLMD
Cannabis Dispensary
Area: Valley Village
Address: 12458 Magnolia Blvd
Valley Village, CA 91607
Phone: (818) 761-9581

#288
Cali Greens
Cannabis Dispensary
Area: San Pedro
Address: 1903 S Pacific
Los Angeles, CA 90731
Phone: (323) 521-3319

#289
Medical Marijuana Delivery Service
Cannabis Dispensary
Area: Redondo Beach
Address: 4001 Inglewood Ave
Redondo Beach, CA 90278
Phone: (424) 209-9333

#290
Beach Side Collective
Cannabis Dispensary
Area: Venice
Address: 1325 Venice Blvd
Venice, CA 90291
Phone: (424) 500-2312

#291
Reliable Relief Collective
Cannabis Dispensary
Area: Woodland Hills
Address: 21777 Ventura Blvd
Woodland Hills, CA 91364
Phone: (818) 881-4420

#292
Sherman Oaks Collective Care
Cannabis Dispensary
Area: Sherman Oaks
Address: 14200 Ventura Blvd
Sherman Oaks, CA 91423
Phone: (818) 783-8332

#293
Beach Center
Cannabis Dispensary
Area: Harbor Gateway
Address: 1115 W 190th
Torrance, CA 90278
Phone: (310) 821-4420

#294
Total Herbal Consultation
Cannabis Dispensary
Area: North Hollywood
Address: 4942 Vineland Ave North
Hollywood, CA 91601
Phone: (818) 350-8183

#295
Foothill Caregivers
Cannabis Dispensary
Area: Tujunga
Address: 7502 Foothill Caregivers
Tujunga, CA 91042
Phone: (818) 353-1859

#296
Best Price Evaluations
Cannabis Dispensary
Address: 8023 Pioneer Blvd
Whittier, CA 90606

#297
Wing Hip Fung Herbal & Ginseng
Cannabis Dispensary
Address: 8118 Garvey Ave
Rosemead, CA 91770

#298
Compassionate Caregivers of San Pedro
Cannabis Dispensary
Area: San Pedro
Address: 410 S Gaffey St
Los Angeles, CA 90731
Phone: (310) 732-2109

#299
True Natural Collective
Cannabis Dispensary
Area: Tujunga
Address: 7568 Foothill Blvd
Tujunga, CA 91042
Phone: (818) 951-6400

#300
Santa Fe Compassionate Health Center
Cannabis Dispensary
Address: 13128 Telegraph Rd
Santa Fe Springs, CA 90670

#301
ATS Alternative Therapeutic
Cannabis Dispensary
Address: 5707 Atlantic Ave
Long Beach, CA 90805

#302
Harbor Area Caregivers Club
Cannabis Dispensary
Area: Harbor Gateway, Torrance
Address: 22708 S Western Ave
Torrance, CA 90501
Phone: (310) 787-9004

#303
DEC
Cannabis Dispensary
Area: Van Nuys
Address: 6309 Van Nuys Blvd
Van Nuys, CA 91401
Phone: (818) 835-1420

#304
New Age Compassion Care Center
Cannabis Dispensary
Area: Hollywood
Address: 1724 N Cahuenga Blvd
Hollywood, CA 90028
Phone: (323) 463-4180

#305
The Nile Collective
Cannabis Dispensary
Area: Venice
Address: 1501 Pacific Ave
Venice, CA 90291
Phone: (310) 392-9900

#306
Ozzys Caregivers
Cannabis Dispensary
Area: Panorama City
Address: 14072 Osborne St
Panorama City, CA 91402
Phone: (818) 830-0320

#307
Az Cancare Collective
Cannabis Dispensary
Area: North Hollywood
Address: 4701 Lankershim Blvd
North Hollywood, CA 91602
Phone: (818) 762-2040

#308
Meds 215
Cannabis Dispensary
Area: Panorama City
Address: 14530 Arminta St
Van Nuys, CA 91402
Phone: (818) 780-5874

#309
Green Earth Farmacie
Cannabis Dispensary
Area: Van Nuys
Address: 6811 Woodman Ave
Van Nuys, CA 91405
Phone: (818) 994-1045

#310
Fast and Friendly
Cannabis Dispensary
Area: Hermosa Beach
Address: 703 Pier Ave
Hermosa Beach, CA 90254
Phone: (310) 870-7115

#311
Ubercollective
Cannabis Dispensary
Area: Beverly Hills
Address: 1234 Mary Jane Ln
Beverly Hills, CA 90212
Phone: (855) 420-8237

#312
The Healing Touch
Cannabis Dispensary
Area: Encino
Address: 18013 Ventura Blvd
Encino, CA 91316
Phone: (818) 881-1462

#313
DC Collective
Cannabis Dispensary
Area: Canoga Park
Address: 8053 Deering Ave.
Canoga Park, CA 91304
Phone: (818) 887-0980

#314
West Valley Caregivers
Cannabis Dispensary
Area: Woodland Hills
Address: 23067 Ventura Blvd
Woodland Hills, CA 91364
Phone: (818) 591-5899

#315
7411 Lankershim Collective
Cannabis Dispensary
Area: Sun Valley
Address: 7411 Lankershim Blvd
North Hollywood, CA 91601
Phone: (818) 764-1203

#316
Green Light District
Cannabis Dispensary
Area: Harbor Gateway
Address: 1635 Carson St
Torrance, CA 90501

#317
Pacific Support Services
Cannabis Dispensary
Area: West Hollywood
Address: 8466 Santa Monica Blvd
West Hollywood, CA 90069
Phone: (877) 468-5874

#318
SCPA
Cannabis Dispensary
Area: Harbor Gateway
Address: 844 W Gardena Blvd
Gardena, CA 90247
Phone: (323) 544-7747

#319
Foothill Wellness Center
Cannabis Dispensary
Area: Tujunga
Address: 7132 Foothill Blvd
Tujunga, CA 91042
Phone: (818) 352-3388

#320
GGR - Gourmet Green Remedies
Cannabis Dispensary
Area: Sawtelle
Address: 2000 Cotner Ave West
Los Angeles, CA 90025
Phone: (310) 473-3509

#321
Automated Medical Group
Cannabis Dispensary
Area: Pacoima
Address: 10568 Kewen Ave
Pacoima, CA 91331
Phone: (818) 834-3673

#322
Collective Care Source
Cannabis Dispensary
Address: 1031 S San Gabriel Blvd
San Gabriel, CA 91776

#323
SFVPG - San Fernando Valley Patients Group
Cannabis Dispensary
Area: Canoga Park
Address: 8244 De Soto Ave
Canoga Park, CA 91304
Phone: (818) 727-0420

#324
Best Price Evaluations
Cannabis Dispensary
Area: Van Nuys
Address: 6819 Sepulveda Blvd
Van Nuys, CA 91405
Phone: (877) 670-6338

#325
1 Love Beach Club
Cannabis Dispensary
Address: 2767 E Broadway
Long Beach, CA 90803

#326
420 Med Mobile
Cannabis Dispensary
Address: S. Atlantic Blvd
Monterey Park, CA 91754

#327
Herbal Solutions Naples
Cannabis Dispensary
Address: 1581 W Wardlow Rd
Long Beach, CA 90810

#328
BEACH Collective Dispensary
Cannabis Dispensary
Area: Harbor Gateway
Address: 1115 W 190th St
Gardena, CA 90248
Phone: (310) 821-4420

#329
Cornerstone Health & Wellness
Cannabis Dispensary
Address: 1838 E Wardlow Rd
Long Beach, CA 90807

#330
Natural Choice Healing Center
Cannabis Dispensary
Area: Valley Glen
Address: 6006 Vantage Ave
North Hollywood, CA 91606
Phone: (818) 358-2620

#331
OMG 2am
Cannabis Dispensary
Address: 11809 E Slauson Ave
Santa Fe Springs, CA 90670

#332
Cure Collective
Cannabis Dispensary
Area: North Hollywood
Address: 10835 Magnolia Blvd
North Hollywood, CA 91601
Phone: (818) 691-3571

#333
Westside Organic Delivery
Cannabis Dispensary
Area: Santa Monica
Address: Santa Monica, CA 90403
Phone: (310) 309-9752

#334
SPAS Medical Marijuana Dispensary
Cannabis Dispensary
Area: San Pedro
Address: 1722 S Gaffey St
San Pedro, CA 90731
Phone: (424) 772-1495

#335
Cannabis Evaluations
Cannabis Dispensary
Area: Pasadena
Address: 50 N Mentor Ave
Pasadena, CA 91106
Phone: (626) 844-5060

#336
Love & Spirit Collective
Cannabis Dispensary
Area: North Hollywood
Address: 5651 1/2 Cahuenga Blvd
North Hollywood, CA 91601
Phone: (818) 753-9200

#337
Alternative Medical Solutions Plus
Cannabis Dispensary
Area: Arleta
Address: 8932 Woodman Ave
Arleta, CA 91331
Phone: (818) 920-6800

#338
So Green Collective
Cannabis Dispensary
Area: Venice
Address: 1325 Venice Blvd
Venice, CA 90291
Phone: (424) 289-9633

#339
Peace Of Green Collective
Cannabis Dispensary
Address: 21720 S Vermont Ave
Torrance, CA 90502

#340
Canna-Centers
Cannabis Dispensary
Address: 15901 Hawthorne Blvd
Lawndale, CA 90260

#341
D.G.R.
Cannabis Dispensary
Area: Tarzana
Address: 18547 Ventura Blvd
Tarzana, CA 91356
Phone: (818) 205-7701

#342
Medical Marijuana Card Doctor
Cannabis Dispensary
Address: 2301 E 28th St
Signal Hill, CA 90755

#343
Venice Beach Physicians
Cannabis Dispensary
Area: Venice
Address: 1825 Ocean Front Walk
Venice, CA 90291
Phone: (310) 741-8878

#344
Daily Care Center
Cannabis Dispensary
Area: North Hollywood
Address: 5430 Cahuenga Blvd
North Hollywood, CA 91601
Phone: (818) 303-6666

#345
NatureCann
Cannabis Dispensary
Address: 4332 Atlantic Ave
Long Beach, CA 90807

#346
Holistic Evaluation
Cannabis Dispensary
Address: 2388 N Lake Ave
Altadena, CA 91001

#347
Sunland Caregivers
Cannabis Dispensary
Area: Sunland
Address: 7831 Foothill Blvd
Sunland, CA 91040
Phone: (818) 951-3344

#348
The Doctor's – Reseda
Medical Marijuana Doctors
Cannabis Dispensary
Area: Reseda
Address: 6650 Reseda Blvd
Reseda, CA 91335
Phone: (818) 654-5882

#349
SFVDM
Cannabis Dispensary
Area: Panorama City
Address: 13550 Roscoe Blvd
Panorama City, CA 91402
Phone: (818) 908-9951

#350
Kester Med Center
Cannabis Dispensary
Area: Van Nuys
Address: 6819 1/2 Kester Ave
Van Nuys, CA 91405
Phone: (818) 945-1135

#351
Canto Diem
Cannabis Dispensary
Area: Studio City
Address: 10612 Chiquita St
North Hollywood, CA 91602
Phone: (818) 821-1209

#352
Green Joy
Cannabis Dispensary
Area: Woodland Hills
Address: 22851 Ventura Blvd
Woodland Hills, CA 91364
Phone: (818) 222-1882

#353
710 Collective
Cannabis Dispensary
Address: 1305 W Willow St
Long Beach, CA 90810

#354
Green Cross
Cannabis Dispensary
Area: Harbor Gateway, Torrance
Address: 1658 W Carson St
Torrance, CA 90501
Phone: (310) 533-9363

#355
PCH Collective
Cannabis Dispensary
Address: 22609 Pacific Coast Hwy
Malibu, CA 90265

#356
Medical Marijuana Evaluation Center
Cannabis Dispensary
Area: Beverly Hills
Address: 8500 Wilshire Blvd
Beverly Hills, CA 90211
Phone: (310) 855-7504

#357
Panorama Providers
Cannabis Dispensary
Area: Panorama City
Address: 13807 Roscoe Blvd
San Fernando Valley, CA 91402
Phone: (818) 894-3300

#358
LabCorp
Cannabis Dispensary
Address: 301 W Huntington Dr
Arcadia, CA 91007

#359
West Valley Patients Group
Cannabis Dispensary
Area: Woodland Hills
Address: 23043 Ventura Blvd
Woodland Hills, CA 91364
Phone: (818) 224-4146

#360
Eden Therapy
Cannabis Dispensary
Area: Hollywood
Address: 6757 Santa Monica Blvd
Hollywood, CA 90038
Phone: (323) 463-8937

#361
Stone Age Pharmacy
Cannabis Dispensary
Area: Harbor Gateway
Address: 621 W. Rosecrans Ave
Gardena, CA 90248
Phone: (310) 366-5906

#362
Puffins
Cannabis Dispensary
Area: Woodland Hills
Address: 23002 Ventura Blvd
Woodland Hills, CA 91364
Phone: (818) 222-7833

#363
Vogc
Cannabis Dispensary
Area: Encino
Address: 17550 Ventura Blvd
Encino, CA 91316
Phone: (818) 398-1559

#364
3PWC
Cannabis Dispensary
Address: 13535 Marquardt Ave
Santa Fe Springs, CA 90670

#365
Delta-9 Torrance Herbal Collective
Cannabis Dispensary
Area: Harbor Gateway
Address: 1321 W. Carson St.
Torrance, CA 90501
Phone: (310) 618-3582

#366
Humboldt Relief
Cannabis Dispensary
Area: Reseda
Address: 6670 Reseda Blvd
Reseda, CA 91335
Phone: (818) 300-0020

#367
Green Dragon
Cannabis Dispensary
Area: Valley Glen
Address: 7236 Varna Ave
North Hollywood, CA 91605
Phone: (818) 442-0054

#368
Connoisseurs League
Cannabis Dispensary
Address: 16510 S Vermont Ave
Gardena, CA 90247

#369
Robertson Caregivers
Cannabis Dispensary
Area: Beverlywood
Address: 2515 S Robertson Blvd
Los Angeles, CA 90034
Phone: (310) 837-7279

#370
Marijuana Market
Cannabis Dispensary
Area: Redondo Beach
Address: 1 Ave A Redondo Beach,
CA 90277
Phone: (310) 272-9074

#371
Beach City Center Solutions
Cannabis Dispensary
Area: Wilmington
Address: 748 N Fries Ave
Wilmington, CA 90744
Phone: (310) 816-0908

#372
Belmont Shore Natural Care
Cannabis Dispensary
Address: 5375 E 2nd St
Long Beach, CA 90803

#373
SCI Sylmar Caregivers
Cannabis Dispensary
Area: Shadow Hills
Address: 9960 Glenoaks Blvd
Sun Valley, CA 91352
Phone: (818) 768-2817

#374
The Hills Collective
Cannabis Dispensary
Area: Woodland Hills
Address: 20000 Ventura Blvd
Woodland Hills, CA 91364
Phone: (818) 999-3265

#375
Green Gorilla Collective
Cannabis Dispensary
Area: Harbor Gateway
Address: 1350 W 228th St
Torrance, CA 90501
Phone: (424) 250-9086

#376
LBC 420 Evaluations
Cannabis Dispensary
Address: 1737 E 7th St
Long Beach, CA 90813

#377
Kush House Caregivers
Cannabis Dispensary
Address: 1213 S Western Ave
Anaheim, CA 92804

#378
**North Hollywood
Compassionate Caregivers**
Cannabis Dispensary
Area: North Hollywood
Address: 4854 Lankershim Blvd
North Hollywood, CA 91601
Phone: (818) 980-9212

#379
Organic Way Collective
Cannabis Dispensary
Address: 13848 E Rosecrans Ave
Santa Fe Springs, CA 90670

#380
Eco Rx
Cannabis Dispensary
Area: North Hollywood
Address: 11428 Vanowen St
North Hollywood, CA 91605
Phone: (818) 358-4490

#381
**North Hollywood
Compassionate Caregivers**
Cannabis Dispensary
Area: North Hollywood
Address: 4854 Lankershim Blvd North
Hollywood, CA 91601
Phone: (818) 980-9212

#382
Ventura Medical Doctors
Cannabis Dispensary
Area: Tarzana
Address: 18346 Ventura Blvd
Tarzana, CA 91356
Phone: (818) 881-5001

#383
**Pasadena Medical Marijuana
Vaporizer Supply**
Cannabis Dispensary
Area: Pasadena
Address: 1224 E Green St
Pasadena, CA 91106
Phone: (626) 219-0644

#384
AP Natural Solutions
Cannabis Dispensary
Address: 9841 Alburtis Ave
Santa Fe Springs, CA 90670

#385
The Source
Cannabis Dispensary
Address: 17421 S Pioneer Blvd
Artesia, CA 90701

#386
Infinity Medical Alliance
Cannabis Dispensary
Area: Harbor Gateway
Address: 1609 Lockness Pl
Torrance, CA 90501
Phone: (310) 891-2223

#387
So Cal Co-op
Cannabis Dispensary
Area: Tarzana
Address: 19459 Ventura Blvd
Tarzana, CA 91356
Phone: (818) 344-7622

#388
South Bay Collective
Cannabis Dispensary
Area: Harbor City
Address: 1151 W. Pacific Coast Hwy
Harbor City, CA 90710
Phone: (310) 530-1628

#389
Zen Medical Garden
Cannabis Dispensary
Area: Tarzana
Address: 18957 Ventura Blvd
Tarzana, CA 91356
Phone: (818) 708-3179

#390
House Of Clones
Cannabis Dispensary
Area: Van Nuys
Address: 7826 Balboa Blvd
Van Nuys, CA 91406
Phone: (818) 988-9907

#391
Willow - Long Beach Natural Solutions
Cannabis Dispensary
Address: 726 W Willow St
Long Beach, CA 90806

#392
LBC 420 Evaluations
Cannabis Dispensary
Address: 720 E Alamitos
Long Beach, CA 90813

#393
Green Earth Pharmacy
Cannabis Dispensary
Area: Van Nuys
Address: 6811 Woodman Ave
Van Nuys, CA 91405
Phone: (818) 994-1045

#394
Go Green Medical Marijuana Dispensary
Cannabis Dispensary
Address: 12145 Slauson Ave
Santa Fe Springs, CA 90670

#395
Sherman Oaks Group Collective SOGC
Cannabis Dispensary
Area: Encino
Address: 15445 Ventura Blvd #8
Sherman Oaks, CA 91403
Phone: (818) 981-1035

#396
Tops Cannabis
Cannabis Dispensary
Address: 964 E Badillo St
Covina, CA 91724

#397
Doctor Green Meds
Cannabis Dispensary
Area: Valley Village
Address: 4741 Laurel Canyon Blvd
Valley Village, CA 91607
Phone: (818) 985-4020

#398
Affordable Evaluations
Cannabis Dispensary
Address: 1040 Elm Ave
Long Beach, CA 90813

#399
ABC Collective Long Beach
Cannabis Dispensary
Address: 5318 E 2nd St
Long Beach, CA 90803

#400
SoCal 420 Doctor Medical Marijuana
Cannabis Dispensary
Address: 4195 Viking Way
Long Beach, CA 90808

#401
Lighthouse Remedy
Cannabis Dispensary
Area: Sylmar
Address: 13127 San Fernando Rd
Sylmar, CA 91342
Phone: (818) 364-7177

#402
Chronic Pain Releaf Center
Cannabis Dispensary
Address: 1501 Santa Fe Ave
Long Beach, CA 90813

#403
Tristar Caregivers
Cannabis Dispensary
Area: Canoga Park
Address: 7211 Owensmouth Ave
Canoga Park, CA 91303
Phone: (818) 887-8653

#404
PR Collective
Cannabis Dispensary
Area: San Pedro
Address: 136 S Gaffey St
San Pedro, CA 90731
Phone: (310) 832-2420

#405
Starlight 420 Center
Cannabis Dispensary
Address: 16540 Leffingwell Rd
Whittier, CA 90603

#406
420 Caregivers
Cannabis Dispensary
Address: 231 N Brookhurst St
Anaheim, CA 92801

#407
Valley Patients
Cannabis Dispensary
Area: Panorama City
Address: 8951 Woodman Ave
Arleta, CA 91331
Phone: (818) 895-5645

#408
Azusa Patient Remedies
Cannabis Dispensary
Address: 393 S Azusa Ave
La Puente, CA 91744

#409
Lake Balboa Collective
Cannabis Dispensary
Area: Lake Balboa
Address: 17616 Sherman Way
Van Nuys, CA 91406
Phone: (818) 514-6374

#410
WEEDeliver Westside
Cannabis Dispensary
Area: Santa Monica
Address: 405 Fwy Santa Monica,
CA 90404
Phone: (424) 744-7777

#411
Focus Relief
Cannabis Dispensary
Area: Panorama City
Address: 8247 1/2 Sepulveda Blvd
Panorama City, CA 91402
Phone: (818) 891-1010

#412
Herbal Solutions
Cannabis Dispensary
Address: 1512 E Broadway St
Long Beach, CA 90802

#413
Healing Tree Holistic Association
Cannabis Dispensary
Address: 3751 E Anaheim St
Long Beach, CA 90804

#414
Beach Medical Center
Cannabis Dispensary
Address: 17822 Beach Blvd
Huntington Beach, CA 92647

#415
Affordabowl
Cannabis Dispensary
Area: North Hollywood
Address: 5645 Cahuenga Blvd
North Hollywood, CA 91601
Phone: (818) 358-3445

#416
American Green Leaf
Cannabis Dispensary
Address: 3011 W Ball Rd
Anaheim, CA 92804

#417
First Choice Wellness
Cannabis Dispensary
Area: San Pedro
Address: 522 W 9th St
San Pedro, CA 90731
Phone: (800) 513-1615

#418
TLC - Toluca Lake Collective
Cannabis Dispensary
Area: North Hollywood
Address: 11436 Hatteras St.
North Hollywood, CA 91601
Phone: (818) 752-8420

#419
Valley Independent Pharmacy
Cannabis Dispensary
Area: Sherman Oaks
Address: 13650 Burbank Bl
Sherman Oaks, CA 91401
Phone: (818) 997-1787

#420
Mid Wilshire Industrial Dispensary
Cannabis Dispensary
Area: Koreatown, Wilshire Center
Address: 3240 Wilshire Blvd Suite 270
Los Angeles, CA 90010
Phone: (213) 507-7530

#421
7 Points Medical
Cannabis Dispensary
Address: 3111 W Ornage Ave
Anaheim, CA 92804

#422
$50 Cap
Cannabis Dispensary
Address: 1066 E Anaheim St
Long Beach, CA 90813

#423
Zen Medical Garden
Cannabis Dispensary
Area: Tarzana
Address: 18957 Ventura Blvd
Tarzana, CA 91356
Phone: (818) 708-3179

#424
On Deck Cooperative
Cannabis Dispensary
Address: 23110 Valencia Blvd
Valencia, CA 91355

#425
Garden Grove Alternative Care
Cannabis Dispensary
Address: 8721 Garden Grove Blvd.
Garden Grove, CA 92844

#426
OrganaCann Wellness Center
Cannabis Dispensary
Address: 12761 Western Ave
Garden Grove, CA 92841

#427
Sticky Leafs Collective
Cannabis Dispensary
Address: 410 S Euclid St
Anaheim, CA 92802

#428
Canna Dispensary of Garden Grove
Cannabis Dispensary
Address: 9758 Chapman Ave
Garden Grove, CA 92841

#429
The Cannaverse
Cannabis Dispensary
Area: San Pedro
Address: 624 W 9th St
San Pedro, CA 90731
Phone: (310) 221-7676

#430
Ocean Shores
Cannabis Dispensary
Address: 2746 E Broadway
Long Beach, CA 90803

#431
Harbor Caregivers
Cannabis Dispensary
Area: Wilmington
Address: 533 N Avalon Blvd
Wilmington, CA 90744
Phone: (310) 830-0144

#432
Green Magic Collective
Cannabis Dispensary
Area: Woodland Hills
Address: 23002 Ventura Blvd
Woodland Hills, CA 91364
Phone: (818) 914-4371

#433
Zen OC
Cannabis Dispensary
Address: 910 Euclid St
Anaheim, CA 92802

#434
Disabled Patients Group
Cannabis Dispensary
Address: 2016 E Anaheim St
Long Beach, CA 90804

#435
Clone Queen Genetics
Cannabis Dispensary
Address: 5152 Katella Ave
Los Alamitos, CA 90720

#436
Affordable Evaluations
Cannabis Dispensary
Address: 431 N Brookhurst St
Anaheim, CA 92801

#437
Euclid Medical Center
Cannabis Dispensary
Address: 12079 S Euclid St
Garden Grove, CA 92840

#438
Green Blossom Medical Dispensary
Cannabis Dispensary
Address: Huntington Beach, CA 92648

#439
HLA Collective
Cannabis Dispensary
Area: Van Nuys
Address: 7123 Sepulveda Blvd
Van Nuys, CA 91405
Phone: (818) 453-8085

#440
Help & Care Center CHC
Cannabis Dispensary
Address: 3702 E Anaheim
Long Beach, CA 90804

#441
Green Guild
Cannabis Dispensary
Address: 26302 Western Ave
Lomita, CA 90717

#442
Aram Wellness Center
Cannabis Dispensary
Address: 9210 Katella Ave
Garden Grove, CA 92841

#443
Open Care Medical Center
Cannabis Dispensary
Address: 2001 E 4th St
Santa Ana, CA 92705

#444
Anaheim Herbal Healing Center
Cannabis Dispensary
Address: 126 N Brookhurst St
Anaheim, CA 92801

#445
Long Beach Quality Discount Caregivers
Cannabis Dispensary
Address: 1150 East San Antonio Dr.
Long Beach, CA 90807

#446
CannaMed of Thousand Oaks
Cannabis Dispensary
Address: 60 N Rancho Rd
Thousand Oaks, CA 91362

#447
Kush Box
Cannabis Dispensary
Address: 12105 Garden Grove Blvd
Garden Grove, CA 92843

#448
Six Seasons
Cannabis Dispensary
Address: Beach & Warner Ave
Garden Grove, CA 92841

#449
40 Healing Patients Center
Cannabis Dispensary
Address: 700 S Euclid St
Anaheim, CA 92802

#450
Aurora Charter Oak Hospital
Cannabis Dispensary
Address: 1161 E Covina Blvd
Covina, CA 91724

#451
California Patients Association
Cannabis Dispensary
Address: 1201 E 17th St
Santa Ana, CA 92701

#452
Medical Marijuana Doctors Anaheim
Cannabis Dispensary
Address: 9774 Katella Ave
Anaheim, CA 92804

#453
Medical Marijuana Doctors
Cannabis Dispensary
Address: 12570 Brookhust St
Garden Grove, CA 92840

#454
Organix Wellness Center
Cannabis Dispensary
Address: 1640 E First St
Santa Ana, CA 92701

#455
Green Hills Patients Association
Cannabis Dispensary
Address: 13311 Garden Grove Blvd
Garden Grove, CA 92843

#456
Pacific Island Care
Cannabis Dispensary
Address: 13071 Brookhurst St
Garden Grove, CA 92843

#457
My Green Fast
Cannabis Dispensary
Address: 1439 W Chapman Ave
Orange, CA 92868

#458
New South Coast Patient Center
Cannabis Dispensary
Address: 1202 E 17th St
Santa Ana, CA 92701

#459
420 Med Pros
Cannabis Dispensary
Address: 1651 E Edinger Ave
Santa Ana, CA 92705

#460
PSA
Cannabis Dispensary
Address: 1536 E Warner Ave
Santa Ana, CA 92705

#461
Med Ex
Cannabis Dispensary
Address: Anaheim, CA 92805

#462
Base Camp Herbal Co-operative
Cannabis Dispensary
Address: 55 Fwy Irvine, CA 92606

#463
Supplemental Organic Solutions
Cannabis Dispensary
Area: Venice
Address: 328 S Lincoln Blvd
Venice, CA 90291
Phone: (310) 450-9141

#464
Cafe Meds
Cannabis Dispensary
Address: 1002 E 17th St
Santa Ana, CA 92701

#465
The Green Machine
Cannabis Dispensary
Address: Malibu, CA 90265

#466
45 Cap
Cannabis Dispensary
Address: 1535 E 17th St
Santa Ana, CA 92705

#467
SoCal Compassion
Cannabis Dispensary
Address: 1651 E Edinger St
Santa Ana, CA 92705

#468
4th Street Medical
Cannabis Dispensary
Address: 2112 E 4th St
Santa Ana, CA 92705

#469
Rollingreens Delivery
Cannabis Dispensary
Address: Santa Ana, CA 92704

#470
Best Price Evaluations
Cannabis Dispensary
Address: 808 N Garey Ave
Pomona, CA 91767

#471
Kush Kingdom
Cannabis Dispensary
Address: 2201-A W 1st St
Santa Ana, CA 92703

#472
Aloha Community Collective Association
Cannabis Dispensary
Address: 1615 N French St
Santa Ana, CA 92701

#473
PSM Professional Safe Meds
Cannabis Dispensary
Address: 1848 W 11th St
Upland, CA 91786

#474
Tops Cannabis
Cannabis Dispensary
Address: 24901 Alicia Pkwy
Laguna Hills, CA 92653

#475
Paragon
Cannabis Dispensary
Address: 1518 N Broadway
Santa Ana, CA 92706

#476
Releaf On 17th
Cannabis Dispensary
Address: 1638 E 17th St
Santa Ana, CA 92705

#477
American Collective
Cannabis Dispensary
Address: 1823 E 17th St
Santa Ana, CA 92705

#478
Epion Medical Centers
Cannabis Dispensary
Address: 1820 E Garry Ave
Santa Ana, CA 92705

#479
Mendica Caregiver
Cannabis Dispensary
Area: Sherman Oaks
Address: Sherman Oaks, CA 91403
Phone: (818) 789-0420

#480
Santa Ana Patient Group
Cannabis Dispensary
Address: 1823 E 17th St
Santa Ana, CA 92705

#481
Advanced Biomedical Cannabis Cooperative
Cannabis Dispensary
Address: 13139 Brookhurst St
Garden Grove, CA 92843

#482
Costa Mesa 420 Evaluations
Cannabis Dispensary
Address: 779 W 19th St
Costa Mesa, CA 92627

#483
The Dispensary Patient Association
Cannabis Dispensary
Address: 1805 E Garry Ave
Santa Ana, CA 92701

#484
Canna-Centers
Cannabis Dispensary
Address: 400 S Ramona Ave
Corona, CA 92879

#485
Canna Care Collective
Cannabis Dispensary
Address: 1638 E 17th St
Santa Ana, CA 92705

#486
215 Agenda
Cannabis Dispensary
Address: 24601 Raymond Way
Lake Forest, CA 92630

#487
Orange County's Patient Care
Cannabis Dispensary
Address: 1921 E Carnegie
Santa Ana, CA 92705

#488
Green Mile Cllective
Cannabis Dispensary
Address: 1823 E 17th St
Santa Ana, CA 92705

#489
Hybrid House Collective
Cannabis Dispensary
Area: Tujunga
Address: 10900 Plainview Ave
Sunland, CA 91042
Phone: (818) 570-4193

#490
Riverside Quality Discount Caregivers
Cannabis Dispensary
Address: 10752 Limonite Ave
Mira Loma, CA 91752

#491
Patients First Cooperative
Cannabis Dispensary
Address: 3503 Interstate 15
Business Lp Norco, CA 92860

#492
So Cal Patients Collective Dispensary
Cannabis Dispensary
Address: 26234 Enterprise Ct
Lake Forest, CA 92630

#493
Unit D
Cannabis Dispensary
Address: 11471 Brookhurst St
Garden Grove, CA 92840

#494
The City 420 Doctor
Cannabis Dispensary
Address: 949 East Palmdale Blvd
Palmdale, CA 93550

#495
Clone Queen Genetics
Cannabis Dispensary
Address: 8516 Vineyard Ave
Rancho Cucamonga, CA 91730

#496
Care Healing Center
Cannabis Dispensary
Address: 2428 Newport Blvd
Costa Mesa, CA 92627

#497
True Holistics
Cannabis Dispensary
Address: 24360 Aphena Ave
Mission Viejo, CA 92691

#498
GGECO
Cannabis Dispensary
Address: 26730 Towne Centre Dr
Foothill Ranch, CA 92610

#499
Lake Forest Designated Caregivers
Cannabis Dispensary
Address: 24602 Raymond Way
Lake Forest, CA 92630

#500
Rite Greens
Cannabis Dispensary
Address: 1801 E Edinger Ave
Santa Ana, CA 92705

www.ingramcontent.com/pod-product-compliance
Lightning Source LLC
Chambersburg PA
CBHW051300170526
45165CB00004B/1796